Choose HEALTH

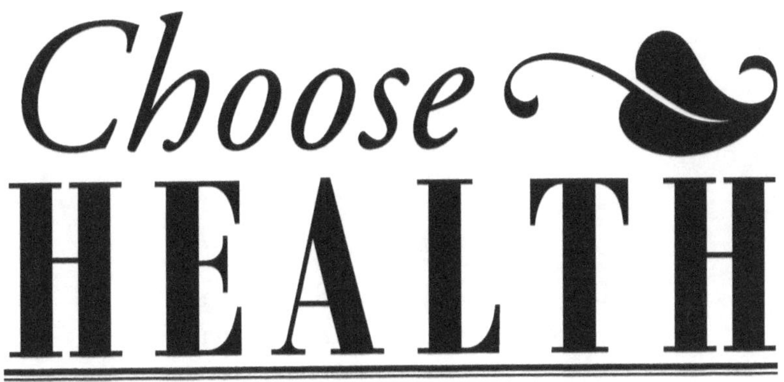

Understanding Prevention and Remedies for Some Common Health Problems

Ifeoma Margaret Ama MD., MPH

Foreword by
Archibald "Chip" Carson, MD, PhD

ISBN 978-1-64471-111-8 (Paperback)
ISBN 978-1-64471-112-5 (Digital)

Covenant Books, Inc.
11661 Hwy 707
Murrells Inlet, SC 29576
www.covenantbooks.com

PREFACE

"Dear friend, I pray that you may enjoy good health and that all may go well with you, even as your soul is getting along well" (3 John 1:2, NIV). This verse shows that God is interested in our being healthy, both in our body and in our soul. Hosea 4:6 says, "My people are destroyed from lack of knowledge" (NIV). It is true that some health conditions don't entirely depend on the actions of people, but there are so many health conditions that can be avoided with the correct information. In my years of medical practice, I have witnessed countless people suffer, and some others die untimely because of circumstances that could have been avoided if they had the right information at their fingertips.

The purpose of this book is to give the readers a basic understanding of some common health issues as well as actions that can be taken to prevent them. The contents of this book should by no means replace optimal medical care including periodic health screening, where applicable.

This book does not provide an exhaustive discussion of the various conditions described. For more detailed information, the *Index* section lists easy-to-find resources where readers can get more information.

The book is divided into three sections. The first section explains the top ten causes of death in the world. The next section explains two diseases that have been in the news over the past few years, Ebola and influenza. The last section presents ten basic actions that one can take to build resistance to diseases and live a healthy and happy life.

CONTENTS

FOREWORD

We, the humans who populate this planet, are its masters, yet we are all victims of the limitations of our bodies and the stress we put on them by our lifestyle choices. We live in an age of progress, of conquering the scourges of the past, of modern technologies and longer life expectancies, and the eradication of the infectious diseases that once ravaged our communities. However, that same progress has brought lifestyle changes and social demands that attack our good health, and an older population that is more susceptible to the chronic diseases associated with ageing. These are now the "common health problems" that are the subject of this book and which are the new leading causes of death and disability in our world.

Dr. Ama intends the following chapters to bring the serious issues of our health and wellness into a personal and easy to understand little book. The vignettes presented here are recognizable to us all and are based upon sound medical advice. They are both entertaining and informative. Readers will gain a new appreciation of their own roles in protecting and promoting the health of their loved ones and themselves.

I was delighted to be asked to provide this opening note. I have known Dr. Ama for several years, first as my graduate student in public health, then as a medical resident, and now as a professional colleague. I have the utmost respect for her as a person, a physician, a wife, and a mother. I admire her concern for her patients and her ability to explain complex medical diagnoses in ways that are easy for her patients to grasp. She is a person of strong faith and commitment; one who, with the help of our creator, achieves the goals she sets for herself. When she told me about this project, I encouraged her to proceed, knowing that the result would educate, improve quality of life, and save people's lives.

So, I encourage you to turn the page, immerse yourself in the drama now unfolding all around you, and become an active participant in the renewal of health and wellbeing in your own life, your family, and your community.

—Archibald "Chip" Carson, MD, PhD

INTRODUCTION

According to the World Health Organization (WHO), the top ten causes of death in the world are ischemic heart disease; stroke; chronic obstructive pulmonary disease; lower respiratory infections; dementias like Alzheimer's disease; cancers of the trachea, lung, and bronchus; diabetes mellitus; road injury; diarrheal diseases; and tuberculosis.

In the United States, the top ten causes of death are heart disease, cancer, chronic lower respiratory diseases, accidents (unintentional injuries), stroke, Alzheimer's disease, diabetes, influenza and pneumonias, kidney diseases, and suicide.

The causes of most deaths in developing countries are mainly cardiovascular disease and infectious diseases, while the causes of most deaths in developed countries are mainly chronic diseases that are caused by unhealthy lifestyle. The aim of this book is to give a basic description of the ten common causes of death, as well as preventive measures that can be taken to prevent these diseases or prevent complications arising where they are already present.

Medical facts can sometimes be technical to the point where understanding the concepts become difficult. This book uses fictional characters to illustrate these health issues to make the learning experience an interesting one. Each chapter starts with a story, breaks up and gives some facts about the health issue being discussed, and then finishes up the story.

The facts and data presented in this book are current at the time of this publication.

SECTION 1

Top Ten Causes of
Death in the World

CHAPTER 1

Isaac, the Executive

Isaac was a top executive in a very successful international investment company. He had started with this company twenty years ago after he moved over from a similar company that was not doing as well as this one. Isaac always referred to himself as a "go-getter." He grew up in a very humble Christian family and went to church three times every week with his parents. He had tried to boycott church as a teenager, but his father would have none of that. Isaac was not permitted to drink alcohol or smoke cigarettes like some of his teenage friends were doing, and he felt like he was in a prison. He was a rational person and was still grateful to his parents for working so hard to care for him and his four siblings.

Isaac was very intelligent and was given a scholarship to go to college in a different state. He was really excited and resolved in his heart to do everything he was unable to do while in "his father's prison" as he referred to his house. His father had given him "the talk" before he left, encouraging him to continue in the way he had been brought up, and Isaac had endured it.

The years had gone by so fast; he had graduated college on top of his class and earned a degree in business. He was immediately hired in an investment company with a fat paycheck. While in college, Isaac had started smoking and drinking, and it had become a habit for him. He even tried illicit drugs but did not like the way they made him feel and didn't continue with the drugs.

It was his forty-fifth birthday, and he decided that he might finally consider getting married. He had not seen his doctor in years as he got tired of being "harassed" to stop smoking, lose weight, and stop drinking. Maybe he would even make an appointment to see his doctor with all the talk in his company about "healthy workforce." He had also been having some chest pressure and occasional shortness of breath when walking the short distance to his favorite burger place. Unfortunately, Isaac did not know that he would be seeing his doctor much sooner than he had planned.

For his birthday, Isaac had invited some friends over for a small party in his beautiful and expensive penthouse. He wanted to use the opportunity to show off his new house to his friends. During the party, he noticed that the chest pressure he had been having for some weeks seemed to be more constant and was even becoming painful. He was a little scared but thought to himself that he was too young to have any serious health problems. That was the last thing he remembered before he found himself in the hospital.

Facts about Ischemic Heart Disease (Heart Attack)

- Over seventeen million people in the world die every year from heart diseases.
- The heart is a vital organ in the body responsible for pumping blood to other parts of the body. The heart is made up of muscles that are also supplied with blood through blood vessels called coronary arteries. Coronary artery disease can lead to inadequate blood flow to the muscles of the heart, leading to a heart attack (also called myocardial infarction).
- Some other types of heart disease include: arrhythmias (when the heart is beating too fast, too slow, or out of rhythm), enlarged heart also known as cardiomegaly, pericarditis (inflammation of the membrane around the heart), endocarditis (inflammation of the inner lining of the heart), and heart failure (when the heart is unable to

pump enough blood to meet the metabolic demands of the body).

- Causes of heart attack include: hypertension, high cholesterol (LDL or bad cholesterol), cigarette smoking, excessive weight, diabetes, excessive alcohol intake, lack of exercise, unhealthy diet.
- Symptoms of heart attack include: chest pain or pressure; pain or discomfort in the arms, back, neck, jaw, or upper abdomen; shortness of breath; nausea; lightheadedness; or cold sweats.
- If you suspect someone is having a heart attack, immediate medical attention is needed. In the emergency room, an EKG (or electrocardiogram, which gives a picture of the electric activity in the heart) can be done; blood tests can also be done to check the levels of the cardiac enzymes; an ultrasound of the heart called an echocardiogram can also be done to aid visualization of the heart, including the force of contraction. If a heart attack is confirmed, prompt medical intervention may avert serious damage to the heart as well as death.
- Complications that could arise from heart attack include: abnormal heart rhythms (arrhythmias), heart failure, damage to the heart muscle, damage to the valves in the heart.
- Heart attack can be prevented by:
- Avoiding cigarette smoking and excessive alcohol intake.
  - Eating at least five servings of fruits and vegetables a day.
  - Limiting salt intake to less than a teaspoon a day.
  - Exercising for at least thirty minutes a day for five days a week.
  - Optimal management of medical conditions like hypertension, high cholesterol, and diabetes by ensuring regular health checks and medication compliance.

Back to Isaac

Dr. Amanda walked in and said, "It's good to finally see you awake, Isaac! We were afraid we were going to lose you. When the ambulance brought you in, you had suffered a heart attack. We immediately took you in for a procedure to restore the blood flow to your heart muscles. You are so lucky that it happened when people were there to call 911. If it had happened while you were sleeping, you might not have made it. By the way, your dad just stepped out to get some food. He looks so young! When he arrived at the hospital very worried yesterday, we thought he was your older brother. The country life seems to suit him well."

Isaac smiled weakly and nodded, he then drifted off into his thoughts. His dad had warned him several times about the danger of the lifestyle he had adopted and he had gotten tired of hearing it, so he refused to go home and he stopped picking up his dad's phone calls. He hadn't spoken with anyone from home in over five years. It was amazing to him that in his time of need, his family was still there for him. He was indeed blessed! God had saved him and given him a second chance. He had abandoned God as well and had stayed away from anything that would remind him of God. He knew he had to find his way back to the God who had indeed been good to him and did not leave him or forsake him. In the midst of his unfaithfulness, God had remained faithful.

What lessons have you learned, and what steps are you willing to take to improve your health?

....

....

....

....

....

....

....

CHAPTER 2

Sarah, the Loving Mom

It was Christmas and everyone was in very high spirits. They had opened gifts and were all very excited to gather around the table to have lunch. This was a very special time for the family. Sarah looked with delight at her family. Her three children, Mark, Abel, and Andrew, had come with their families for the holiday. This was a special time, for her home had grown very cold since her children had grown up and moved out to start families of their own. Her husband had died almost ten years before, due to a work-related accident, and she had worked very hard to cater to her family as a single parent. She spent most of her spare time gardening and attending events in her church. The community had been there for her since her husband had died, and she was very grateful for all the help she had received.

She was so lost in her thoughts that she didn't hear Mark call out to her. "Mom!" Mark called out again. "We are ready to pray. We don't want the delicious meal you have prepared to get cold." Sarah smiled and began to pray. As they started eating, Sarah called out to Abel. "Abe!"—as she fondly called him, "Could you please pass the salt to me?" "Yes, Mom," he replied and passed it over to her. There was a loud *thud* as the saltshaker dropped on the glass table. That was when Abel noted that Sarah's face seemed to be deviated to the left side. "Mom, are you alright?" Abel called out. Sarah tried to respond but couldn't seem to get the words out. Then Abel ran to her side and held her, while shouting to Mark to call 911.

Everything seemed to happen so quickly from then on. Within the next few minutes, they were all in the waiting area of the emergency room of their community hospital. The doctor came out and told them that their mother had suffered an ischemic stroke, which happened because a blood clot had blocked blood flow to a part of her brain. He explained to them that because they came to the hospital very quickly, their mom was a good candidate for a medication called "tissue plasminogen activator." They were all very grateful to God that this had happened when they were with her and not when she was alone.

Facts about Stroke

- Stroke is the second leading cause of death and claims over six million lives globally every year.
- A stroke occurs when there is interruption in the blood supply to a part of the brain.
- There are two types of stroke:
  - Ischemic stroke occurs when there is a blockage to one or more arteries that supply blood to the brain.
  - Hemorrhagic stroke is said to have occurred when there is damage to a blood vessel in the brain, causing bleeding in the brain.
- Causes of stroke include cigarette smoking, alcohol abuse, lack of exercise, high cholesterol, diabetes, hypertension, excessive salt intake.
- The brain controls many different functions in the body, therefore the symptoms of stroke will depend on the part of the brain that is affected. Symptoms could include difficulty speaking, weakness of the hands or legs, asymmetry of the face, memory problems, difficulty seeing, dizziness, or headache.
- Diagnosis is aided by imaging such as CT scan of the brain and MRI.

- Prompt medical attention should be sought for people who are suspected to have strokes, because early intervention may prevent further brain damage. Trained medical professionals can perform procedures to either remove the clot or repair the damaged blood vessel in the brain, where possible, depending on the type of stroke.
- In severe cases, stroke could lead to permanent brain damage causing memory impairment, speech impairment, or weakness of the hands or legs.
- Prevention includes maintaining a healthy diet including a low-salt diet, regular exercise, maintaining a healthy weight, avoiding cigarette smoking, optimal management of medical conditions such as high cholesterol, diabetes, and hypertension.

Later that Week…

Sarah was transferred to a rehabilitation facility for treatment of weakness of the right side of her body. She was very motivated and participated in all her rehab sessions. She also attended health education classes at the rehab facility and was very pleased with the amount of knowledge she had gained. Members of her family, as well as her church members, visited her regularly, and she was grateful to have the much needed support. After about three months she had almost completely recovered and was discharged home to the care of her family. She was very excited to go home and commence the healthy lifestyle she had learned while at the rehab facility.

What lessons have you learned, and what steps are you willing to take to improve your health?

CHAPTER 3

Claudia, the Wife of Laban

Claudia noticed that she was getting increasingly short of breath. The last few weeks had been very eventful indeed. Her husband Laban, who had been smoking cigarettes for so many years, had recently done a CT scan of his lungs for lung cancer screening and they were awaiting the results. A few days after the scan, they received the "dreaded" call from their doctor that there were two suspicious growths seen in his lungs. The doctor ordered several blood tests to prepare for a biopsy, which had finally been done after it was rescheduled twice. Claudia had initially attributed her shortness of breath to all the running around, but she also noticed that she had a cough that had lasted for over two months that wasn't going away. She had gone back to her doctor, who sent her to go do a lung function test called a "spirometry." The results of the test showed that she had chronic obstructive pulmonary disease (COPD). Her doctor had informed her that the cause of her disease was most likely "secondhand smoke." This was not the first time she had heard about secondhand smoke. However, the first time she heard about it, her husband Laban had dismissed it as "a scare tactic to pressure people to quit smoking." Unfortunately, she now had to deal with this disease for the rest of her life. Her doctor prescribed some medications for her that were supposed to make her feel better, and told her to return for follow-up in two months.

Facts about Chronic Obstructive Pulmonary Disease (COPD)

- Over sixty-four million people in the world have COPD, and it is the third leading cause of death.
- COPD is a group of diseases that cause airflow obstruction in the lungs and breathing problems.
- It leads to inflammation of the lungs and destruction of the lung structure.
- This disease develops slowly and gets worse over time. It could eventually result in dependence on supplemental oxygen for survival.
- Types of COPD include emphysema and chronic bronchitis.
- Causes include: cigarette smoking, including breathing in secondhand smoke (secondhand smoke is the air that contains cigarette smoke that is inhaled by someone in close proximity to a person who is smoking), prolonged exposure to dust or fumes, infections of the respiratory system, genetic conditions such as alpha-1 antitrypsin deficiency.
- Symptoms include cough that produces lots of mucus, especially first thing in the morning ("smoker's cough"), wheezing, shortness of breath, chest tightness.
- Severe symptoms that require urgent medical evaluation include difficulty talking, bluish fingernails or lips, reduced mental alertness, fast heartbeat, worsening symptoms despite adherence to prescribed medications.
- Diagnosis of COPD is done primarily by physical exam, in conjunction with pulmonary function tests like spirometry. Chest X-ray and CT scan may also show signs of damage to the lungs especially in advanced cases. Blood tests can also be done to check the level of oxygen in the arteries.
- There is currently no cure for COPD, however medications can be given to improve quality of life. Smoking cessation is very important to stop the ongoing damage to the lungs. Medications such as inhalers that help to dilate the

airways, as well as steroids that help to reduce the inflammation, may also be prescribed, depending on the stage of the disease.

- Due to the compromised state of the lungs, COPD patients are susceptible to infections such as flu and pneumonia. It is therefore recommended that people with COPD get vaccinated against these diseases.
- Pulmonary rehabilitation, which involves breathing strategies, exercise training, and nutritional counseling can be done to improve quality of life.
- Oxygen is prescribed for patients in whom the lung function is impaired to the extent that the level of oxygen in the blood is low.
- Surgery, such as lung transplant, can be done on people with very severe disease.
- Complications include difficulty with physical activity such as walking, mental confusion, memory loss, depression, frequent hospitalization, and difficulty maintaining social interactions.
- Prevention of COPD involves avoiding cigarette smoking, including secondhand smoking, avoiding air pollution, including dust and chemical fumes that can irritate the lungs.

Two-Month Follow Up

Two months later, Claudia felt a lot better. Laban had finally quit smoking. They had also done extensive cleaning and remodeling of their house to get rid of the smell of cigarette smoke that had been deposited on their furniture over the years.

Claudia subsequently became an advocate for stopping secondhand smoking. She shared her experience with members of her community and was happy she could help prevent others from going through her ordeal.

What lessons have you learned, and what steps are you willing to take to improve your health?

CHAPTER 4

Pete, the Collector

Pete beamed with joy as he admired his most recent collections. He had gone to an antique show and bought some Victorian chairs that were at least one hundred years old. He planned someday to set up a mini-museum where members of the community could come and learn about various historical items. His rasping cough brought him back to reality. He had been coughing for over a week now, and last night he thought he had a fever. He hadn't gotten around to buying a thermometer; it would have come in handy to check his temperature and know for sure if he had a fever or not. He remembered that he had a prolonged conversation with a woman at the antique show who had also been coughing and looked as if she needed to see a doctor. Could he have gotten some weird infection from her? He decided to have some vegetable soup and get some rest, hoping that he would feel better by the end of the day. Around 8:00 p.m., he was feeling much worse and didn't need a thermometer to know that he had a fever. He decided to go to the emergency room of the community hospital. Upon arrival, he was given a face mask to wear. The nurse told him that it was their protocol to prevent respiratory disease transmission in the waiting room. He didn't mind at all, because he didn't want anyone to fall ill on his account. He didn't wait long before he was taken into a room to be seen by the doctor. After initial evaluation, the doctor sent him for blood tests and a chest X-ray that confirmed he had pneumonia. He was then admitted to an observation unit for treatment with intravenous antibiotics.

Facts about Lower Respiratory Infections

- Pneumonia is the most common lower respiratory infection and it affects about 450 million people in the world annually and causes millions of deaths. Most deaths from pneumonia occur in children less than five years old or adults greater than sixty-five years old.
- Bronchitis and bronchiolitis are also lower respiratory tract infections but are not as common as pneumonia.
- About 50,000 people die from this disease every year in the United States. Although most cases of pneumonia are caused by bacteria, viruses are the culprits in almost half of the cases. Pneumonia can also be caused by fungi.
- When a person has pneumonia, the alveoli (air sacs) in the lungs, which should normally contain air, get inflamed and become filled with pus and fluid. This reduces the amount of oxygen that enters the blood through the lungs and also leads to pain with breathing. The organisms that cause pneumonia can be spread to other people when an infected person coughs or sneezes.
- Types of pneumonia:
  - Community-acquired pneumonia: here, infection is spread from person to person in the community.
  - Healthcare-associated pneumonia: this type of pneumonia is developed during or after staying at a healthcare facility, such as a hospital or dialysis center.
- Anyone can get pneumonia; however, more severe disease occurs in people who have compromised immunity, such as children (especially malnourished children), formula-fed infants, individuals with diabetes, individuals with HIV/AIDS, individuals taking immunosuppressant medications, and adults sixty-five and older. People with

long-standing respiratory problems are also at risk of developing severe pneumonia, such as individuals with asthma or chronic obstructive pulmonary disease. Cigarette smoking, including secondhand smoking (inhaling the air contaminated by cigarette smoke), also compromises the integrity of the lungs and increases the risk of developing severe pneumonia.

- Symptoms include fever, cough, difficulty breathing, and wheezing (especially in viral pneumonia).
- Pneumonia can be diagnosed by a doctor who might order a chest X-ray, sputum analysis, or blood and urine tests.
- Bacterial pneumonia is treated with antibiotics, which may be given in oral form or intravenous form depending on the severity of the disease. Severe cases may warrant hospitalization with oxygen treatment.
- Complications of pneumonia include damage to the lungs, movement of bacteria from the lungs to the blood causing infection in the blood, a condition called "septicemia," and death in severe cases.
- Pneumonia can be prevented by practicing good hygiene, such as staying away from others who are sick, covering the mouth when coughing, and washing hands with soap and water. Also, some of the routine childhood and adult vaccinations help to prevent some types of pneumonia.

Two Days Later

Pete's symptoms had improved significantly after two days of intravenous antibiotics treatment, and he was discharged home on oral antibiotics to complete the treatment. His doctor encouraged him to adhere to the medication instructions in order to prevent resistant bacteria from developing. He was very grateful to feel well again. He had also learned the importance of healthy practices like covering the mouth when coughing and staying away from crowded places when sick. He hoped that he would not have to go through the same experience again.

What lessons have you learned, and what steps are you willing to take to improve your health?

CHAPTER 5

Dinah, the business woman

Dinah was a very accomplished lady. She and her husband, Eli, had started their own business selling groceries in the community, and their business had grown over thirty years. They had been able to pay the full college fees for their four children from the profit they had made from the grocery store. Their children had also enjoyed working at the store during summer holidays and making extra money. Their children were all grown now and had moved to other neighboring cities. However, they maintained a great relationship with their parents and came to see them on a regular basis. Dinah loved walking the short distance from their home to their grocery store, but in the past few months, she had occasionally forgotten how to walk there and had become lost in the neighborhood. She initially passed it off as old age, but Eli had also noticed that she had been making mistakes with the store accounts. He hired an account manager for the store, hoping it would help the situation. Eli didn't think much about the fact that Dinah would often forget the names of their customers, passing it off as "old age." Unfortunately, Dinah's condition seemed to be deteriorating, and they decided that she should go see a medical professional. The visit took a little longer than they had expected. At the end of the visit they were sad to learn that Dinah might be suffering from a form of dementia known as Alzheimer's dementia. They didn't know if either of Dinah's parents had the condition, as she was adopted and did not know anything about her biological parents. They were hopeful when they were informed about an Alzheimer's disease support group that was available to members of their community. From the hospital, they went to register with the support group and received lots of helpful materials.

Facts about Dementia

- About fifty million people in the world have dementia.
- Dementia refers to the loss of mental abilities. It is usually progressive, that is, it gets worse over time. It occurs in both young people and older people but is more common in older people.
- Alzheimer's disease is the most common form of dementia. Another type is vascular dementia.
- Some of the risk factors include: genetic inheritance, tobacco use, excessive alcohol intake, diabetes, hypertension, lack of exercise, unhealthy diet, obesity, and depression.
- Symptoms include: forgetfulness, getting lost easily especially in familiar places, losing track of time, forgetting people's names, communication difficulties, needing help with grooming, asking repetitious questions, difficulty walking, and aggression in severe cases.
- There is no cure for dementia at this time; however, adequate treatment of any underlying medical problem, where possible, would help to prevent further deterioration of brain function. Early diagnosis is important to establish an optimal quality of life.
- **Prevention:**
  - Avoid tobacco use, alcohol abuse, and unhealthy diet.
  - Exercise for at least thirty minutes a day on most days.
  - Disease conditions like diabetes and hypertension should be adequately managed.

One Year Later

Dinah and Eli adjusted their lifestyle and were as happy as they could be. Eli hired a store manager to take care of the store and enjoyed taking daily walks with Dinah around their neighborhood. They had developed a system of posting sticky notes to remind Dinah of various household tasks and Dinah felt less stressed than she previously did. They also contributed generously to the Alzheimer's disease support group and participated in the "Walk to End Alzheimer's Disease." At their follow-up appointments, their doctor was very happy with Dinah's progress and with the support she was getting from Eli and the members of the community.

What lessons have you learned, and what steps are you willing to take to improve your health?

CHAPTER 6

Laban, the loving husband

Laban sat in the doctor's office waiting to be called in for his evaluation prior to surgery. He had been recently diagnosed with early-stage lung cancer. His doctor had previously recommended a CT scan to screen for lung cancer, but Laban was initially doubtful of the relevance of such screening, since he did not have any symptoms suggestive of lung cancer. His wife Claudia had talked him into getting the test done and he had complied. He was happy he listened to his wife and doctor, as the scan picked up early-stage disease. His joy however was dampened by the fact that his lovely wife Claudia had recently been diagnosed with chronic obstructive pulmonary disease (COPD), which was caused by her exposure to tobacco smoke from him for the thirty-three years they had been married. He wished he could turn back the hands of time. What had started as a high school experiment with some of his friends had gone on to become a habit for him. Most of his other friends belonged to a church where smoking was frowned upon, and they had all dropped cigarette smoking. He, on the other hand, didn't go to church or any other religious gathering. He wanted to be able to do whatever he wished without being judged by people.

The nurse called him to come in to see the doctor. "Hello, Laban," Dr. Allen called out to him. "It's great to see you again!" The doctor went on to tell him that all the preoperative screening was fine and that they were on target to do the surgery in two weeks to remove as much of the cancerous tissue from his lungs as they could. The doctor was also pleased to learn that Laban had quit smoking.

Facts about Lung Cancer

- Over eight million people die from various types of cancers in countries all over the world every year.
- Cancer is said to occur when abnormal cells multiply without control. These cells may form "tumors" and invade other organs in the body, causing damage to these organs. When a cancer originates in one organ and spreads to other organs it is said to have metastasized. There are over a hundred types of cancers.
- According to WHO, cancer of the trachea, bronchus, and lungs are collectively among the top ten causes of death in the world. The main risk factor these cancers have in common is cigarette smoking. Of these three cancers, lung cancer is the most common.
- Other risk factors for lung cancer besides cigarette smoking include: secondhand smoking by inhaling the cigarette smoke released into the air by others who are smoking, radon exposure (a naturally occurring colorless and odorless radioactive gas that can enter some houses from the underlying soil), family history, HIV infection, excessive weight, lack of exercise, high-dose radiation exposure, exposure to air pollution, exposure to asbestos, and exposure to some heavy metals such as chromium and arsenic.
- Symptoms of lung cancer include persistent cough, chest pain, shortness of breath, wheezing, coughing up blood, excessive tiredness, and weight loss.
- Diagnosis of lung cancer involves blood tests, respiratory fluid analysis, imaging studies, such as CT scan and lung biopsy (where a small portion of the affected area is taken out and observed under the microscope).

- Treatment of lung cancer depends on the histological type of the cancer (determined by observing the cancer cells under a microscope) and the extent of the disease. Treatment could involve surgery, chemotherapy (medications that kill cancer cells) and/or radiation therapy.
- **Prevention:**
  - Avoid cigarette smoking and secondhand smoking.
  - Where available, test your house for radon.
  - Avoid air pollution and avoid exposure to asbestos and metals known to cause lung cancer.

Two Weeks Later

Laban had a successful surgery. The mass was bigger than they had predicted from the CT scan; however, after six hours of surgery, doctors were able to remove all the cancerous tissue from his lungs. His wife, Claudia, was by his side as usual and stayed with him until he was discharged from the hospital. In the months that followed, Laban had a painful recovery. When he was much better, he joined his wife Claudia to go about giving lectures and seminars, especially to the youth in their community, warning them about the dangers of cigarette smoking.

What lessons have you learned, and what steps are you willing to take to improve your health?

....

....

....

....

....

....

....

....

CHOOSE HEALTH

CHAPTER 7

Dorcas, the Designer

Dorcas had been feeling very tired over the past few months, but she had initially passed it off as her body reacting to stress at work. She worked for a company that was one of the largest suppliers of clothes for adults and children, and over the years she had distinguished herself at work as a talented designer. She had recently won a contract to design the clothes that would be worn by a soccer team for their next tournament. As a result of all the time she was spending at work, she had paid very little attention to her diet. She had resorted to fast food for most of her meals, and she hadn't exercised for a long time. Initially she put on twenty pounds two years ago, and six months later she had gained another thirty pounds. The last time she checked her weight, six months ago, she had gained over eighty pounds, at which point she stopped checking her weight because she did not want to be upset. She didn't even remember the last time she saw her primary care physician for a wellness check. She finally decided to call for an appointment as she had recently turned forty. She also noticed that she had been urinating more frequently and seemed to constantly be thirsty, and her vision had become very blurry. She didn't like to drink water, so she had been drinking sugary beverages when she was thirsty.

Upon arriving at her doctor's office, she was weighed and was shocked that she learned she had gained ninety pounds in two years. She also had some blood work done and was told that she had diabetes. This came as a rude shock to her as she didn't think she would ever have to deal with any chronic disease. In fact, the doctor told her that her blood sugar level was so high that she would need to start daily insulin injections and oral medications, as well as significant lifestyle modifications, including healthy diet and exercise. Dorcas was upset at the thought of having to take daily injections but was motivated when her Doctor told her that if she was able to lose some weight, they might be able to discontinue the injections. She was given an appointment to follow up in three months.

Facts about Diabetes Mellitus

- Diabetes mellitus, simply called diabetes, is a chronic disease caused by impairment in insulin secretion, insulin utilization, or both. Insulin is a hormone that helps to regulate the amount of sugar in the blood. It is produced by an organ in the body called the pancreas.
- There are over 400 million people in the world with diabetes and the disease has caused millions of deaths worldwide.
- Types of diabetes include:
- Type 1 diabetes, in which there is no insulin production, can occur at any age. Insulin replacement is necessary for survival.
    - Type 2 diabetes is the most common type of diabetes and can also occur at any age. Patients with this kind of diabetes still have some insulin production, but there is a problem with insulin utilization by the body. Both insulin and oral medications can be used for treatment of this condition.
    - Gestational diabetes is the type of diabetes that occurs during pregnancy and in most people resolves after delivery.
    - Prediabetes is the stage before a person develops overt diabetes. It is also known as impaired glucose tolerance. This is a critical stage because most people, if dis-

covered at this stage, can avoid progression to diabetes by adopting healthy lifestyle measures.

- People who have other people in their family with diabetes are at a greater risk of having the disease. Cigarette smoking, obesity, and lack of exercise can also predispose an individual to develop diabetes.
- Symptoms include excessive urination, excessive thirst, blurry vision, excessive tiredness, and weight loss in some cases.
- Blood tests can be done to check the level of the sugar in the blood. This includes fasting blood sugar (here an individual is asked to avoid eating anything before the test), random blood sugar (individuals are tested even after they have eaten) and Hemoglobin A1c (gives a picture of the average blood sugar level in the preceding three months; a level greater than or equal to 6.5% is diagnostic of diabetes. A level 5.7 to 6.4% is regarded as prediabetes and a level 4 to 5.6% is normal).
- Possible complications of diabetes include blindness, kidney failure, wound infections leading to amputation of limbs, heart disease, and stroke.
- Steps that can be taken to prevent the onset of diabetes as well as complications from the disease include:
  - Eating a healthy diet comprising of whole grains, proteins, fruits, fish, lean meat, and vegetables, while avoiding excessive sugar and simple carbohydrates.
  - Maintaining a normal body weight: BMI of 18.5 to 24.9 (Body mass index or BMI is calculated by dividing your weight in kilograms by the height in meters squared kg/m^2).
  - Exercising for at least thirty minutes a day for five days a week.
  - Avoiding cigarette smoking.

Follow-Up Appointment

Three months later, Dorcas returned for follow up and had become more intentional about her diet. She had stopped eating fast food and now prepared wholesome meals at home, mostly comprising of vegetables and whole grains. She had also started walking for forty minutes daily for five days a week. She had reviewed her work hours with her supervisor and stopped unnecessary overtime, which allowed her to rest well at night. Her doctor was very impressed when she checked Dorcas's weight and it was forty pounds down from the previous visit. Her blood sugar level had also improved and Dorcas was taken off insulin and asked to continue with the pills alone, as well as healthy lifestyle. Dorcas was delighted. She decided that she was going to continue to work on her new lifestyle and maybe someday she would even be able to get off medications entirely. She also set up a meeting to meet with the mayor of the city to start a free diabetes class for members of the community where they could learn healthy eating habits as well as healthy lifestyle choices. She was determined to continue to make continuous positive progress. Her next appointment was in six months. She couldn't wait to see how her numbers would look on that appointment.

What lessons have you learned, and what steps are you willing to take to improve your health?

....
....
....
....
....
....
....

CHAPTER 8

Rufus, the Programmer

Rufus was a workaholic. He was the first to get to work and the last one to leave. He was a computer programmer and was designing a new computer program for the company. He always tried to finish assigned tasks before the deadline and had been nominated Employee of the Year for five years in a row. Rufus had been working on the computer program all week and wanted to turn in the completed project by Monday. He was not supposed to work at home but he had access to the computer system and decided to complete the project that weekend. On Sunday night, he could finally see the light at the end of the tunnel and he kept going. He completed the project around 2:00 a.m. and barely slept before his alarm went off at 5:00 a.m. He slowly got out of his bed and got ready for work. He was so sleepy that he had worn 2 different colors of socks but he did not notice it. He knew that he was not well rested and he was still tired. He could call a cab to take him to work, but decided to drive instead. He was already halfway to work when he realized that he had forgotten his laptop and had to return home to get it. On his way back, he was struggling to get through the early morning traffic when his phone beeped on the front passenger seat. He looked down quickly and saw that it was a message from his boss. While grabbing the phone to read the message, he heard the loudest noise he could ever remember hearing. He had "T-boned" an oncoming vehicle at an intersection, and all he remembered was seeing shattered glass flying in different directions before he woke up in the intensive care unit.

Facts about Road Traffic Injuries

- More than 1.25 million people die each year from road traffic accidents, and many others suffer permanent disability from these accidents.
- Males are more likely to be involved in road accidents than females.
- Causes of road accidents include speeding, driving under the influence of alcohol, driving under the influence of drugs or medications that cloud memory, motorcycle riding without a helmet, driving or riding in a vehicle without seatbelts, failing to use child restraints, distracted driving (which could be due to use of cell phones while driving), driving when tired with poor concentration, driving on poorly designed roads, driving unsafe vehicles.
- Individuals involved in a road accidents should seek medical attention as soon as possible. Symptoms that may occur immediately after the accident or days after the accident include cuts on the skin, broken bones, head injury, sprains, pain, dizziness, numbness and/or anxiety.
- To prevent road accidents, avoid drinking and driving, avoid using cell phones when driving, do not drive if you are taking medications that could impair mental function (such as medications that have drowsiness as a side effect), and avoid driving when fatigued. Vehicles and roads should be properly maintained.

In the Intensive Care Unit

After Rufus woke up, he was told that the other driver, a forty-two-year-old mother of three, had died on the scene a few minutes after the impact. She was not wearing her seat belt and had been thrown out of her car through the shattered windshield. Rufus was praying that he was dreaming, but he was not. He had been in the hospital for two months and woke up at the point when they thought he was never going to make it. He did not feel lucky at all, he wished he could turn back the hand of time. He should never have driven when he was so tired, and he shouldn't have tried to read a message on his phone while driving. He had always heard about people who were involved in motor vehicle accidents and had even seen car crashes on his way to work on several occasions, but he never imagined that he would be involved in such a devastating situation. It was then that he picked up his phone and read his boss's message that he had started reading two months before which said, "Good morning, Rufus, I will be out of town today. Please take the day off and get some rest." With everything that had happened, his project deadline didn't matter anymore.

What lessons have you learned, and what steps are you willing to take to improve your health?

CHAPTER 9

Darius, the happy toddler

Darius was a very energetic eighteen-month-old boy. He was the only child of his parents, and they loved him very much. He was born in an underdeveloped country where the majority of the people lacked food and potable water. His father worked as a miner in a village that was far away from home and only came back for the weekends. They were hopeful that things would improve. Darry, as he was fondly called, loved to play outside, and he had the biggest smile in their village. For about two days his mum had noticed that he had been passing five loose stools daily and he also had a fever. She had used all the money she had to buy "fever medication," which had only slightly improved his condition. Darry hadn't been eating or playing like he would normally do.

On the third day, his mother was even more concerned and decided to take him to the nearest hospital, which was four hours away. Upon arriving at the emergency room of the hospital, Darry was already severely dehydrated, and unfortunately he died while the medical staff was trying to resuscitate him. His mother's tears were endless. She wished she had come to the hospital sooner than she did. Unfortunately, this was a very common occurrence in this part of the world. Most other children would even die before they get to the hospital.

Facts about Diarrheal Diseases

- There are about 1.7 billion cases of childhood diarrheal diseases every year out of which over 500,000 children die every year.
- Diarrhea is said to occur when an individual has three or more loose bowel movements a day that are different from the individual's usual bowel movement.
- Types of diarrhea include watery diarrhea (cholera), bloody diarrhea (dysentery), and persistent diarrhea (which lasts two weeks or more).
- Diarrhea can be caused by various organisms such as bacteria, viruses, and parasites. People get infected when they eat contaminated food or drink contaminated water and they can pass the infection to others, especially with poor hygiene.
- When diarrhea occurs, prompt medical attention is necessary, especially for persistent diarrhea, severe dehydration, and any blood in the stool.
- Dehydration occurs due to loss of fluid from watery stools and poor oral intake. This could lead to death in affected individuals. Mild dehydration may manifest by excessive thirst. Severe dehydration could lead to restlessness, lethargy, sunken eyes, and unconsciousness.
- Oral rehydration solution (ORS), which is a solution containing water, sugar, and minerals, has prevented lots of deaths from dehydration due to diarrhea. Zinc tablets may also be taken for two weeks.
- Hospitalization with intravenous fluid administration may be necessary in severe dehydration.
- Diarrhea can be prevented by drinking safe water, hand washing with soap, maintaining a clean environment, and getting rotavirus vaccination.

Darius never lived to see his second birthday. He never got to go to school, ride a bicycle, learn to swim, or even see his father again.

If only his mother had known about oral rehydration solution, she would have spent half of the money she had spent and her little boy would have had a better fighting chance.

There was a young physician in the hospital the night Darius died who resolved to reach out to as many people as she can in various communities like Darry's village and educate them on the dangers of dehydration and how to prevent death from dehydration.

What lessons have you learned, and what steps are you willing to take to improve your health?

CHAPTER 10

Tobiah, the researcher

Tobiah had been working on a clinical research project for the past year that mostly involved going out to the community and having the research participants fill out very long questionnaires. He rarely had enough time to eat a wholesome meal, and he was in the habit of skipping meals. So when he noticed that he had lost fifteen pounds in three months, he assumed that it was as a result of his tasking work and poor diet. The project was set to be concluded in three months, at which time he planned to go on a two-week ship cruise. He had also noticed that he had a stubborn cough that refused to go away despite all the over-the-counter cough medications he had been taking. He finally decided to seek medical attention.

He arrived at the doctor's office where he was given a face mask to wear, upon reporting his symptoms. He felt that they were over-reacting but just decided to play along. After ten minutes, he was called in to a room to see the doctor. After explaining his symptoms to his doctor, a chest X-ray was performed in the clinic, which was highly suggestive of tuberculosis. He also submitted sputum samples for analysis to confirm the diagnosis.

How could this have happened, he asked himself. His doctor told him not to feel bad, as one in four people in the world have been exposed to tuberculosis and have the tuberculosis bacteria in their bodies. Most people's immune system is strong enough to contain the disease for very long periods of time, until such a time as something happens to weaken the immune system, at which time the tuberculosis disease becomes active. His doctor went on to explain that his poor diet and stressful work conditions must have reduced his immunity, making him susceptible to tuberculosis disease. He was then assured that medications were available to treat the disease, but that he should be very compliant with the medications, as non-compliance could lead to the emergence of multidrug-resistant TB. He was going to take the medications for nine months.

Facts about Tuberculosis

About two billion people in the world are infected with tuberculosis (TB) and 1.7 million people in the world died from TB in 2016.

- Tuberculosis is caused by a type of bacterium called Mycobacterium tuberculosis that causes damage mostly to the lungs, but can also affect the kidney, spine, brain, and other organs.
- A type of tuberculosis that is resistant to the usual drugs used to treat the disease has emerged over the years called multidrug-resistant TB and this is currently a public health crisis.
- Types of tuberculosis:
  - Latent tuberculosis infection is the form that exists in most infected people. These people may have been exposed to the disease at some point, but do not have any symptoms of tuberculosis.
  - Active tuberculosis or TB disease is the form of tuberculosis where the infected person has symptoms and can transmit the disease to other people.
- The disease is usually spread when a person with TB disease coughs or speaks, releasing bacteria into the air. When this infected air is breathed by others, they may become

infected. Not everyone who is infected goes on to develop TB disease.

- Some of the factors that lead to the development of TB disease include long-standing diseases of the lungs and immunosuppression that may be caused by HIV infection, substance abuse, severe kidney disease, diabetes mellitus, low body weight, organ transplant, and use of some medications that can weaken the immune system, for example, steroids.

- Symptoms of TB disease may include cough lasting three weeks or more, occasional blood in the sputum, chest pain, fever, night sweats, weakness, feeling unwell, loss of appetite, and weight loss.

- Diagnosis is by tuberculosis skin testing, sputum analysis, blood tests, chest X-ray.

- TB disease and latent tuberculosis can both be treated with medications that kill the bacteria causing the disease in most cases. It is important to adhere to the treatment regimen to prevent further emergence of resistant strains of the bacteria.

- If left untreated, TB disease could lead to death. Other possible complications include damage to the lungs and predisposition to uncommon fungal infections in the lungs.

- **Prevention**
  - When an individual has symptoms suggestive of TB, early diagnosis and initiation of treatment helps to prevent its spreading to other people.
  - Practice good hygiene such as covering of cough and sneezes.
  - Indoor environments should be well ventilated and well lit.
  - Infected people should stay away from others until advised by a healthcare professional that they are no longer infectious. Although the treatment of tuberculosis takes several months to complete, about two to

four weeks after starting treatment most people will no longer be infectious.

- ○ Healthcare workers should be screened regularly for latent tuberculosis and treated if they are found to be positive.
- ○ Individuals should be screened for latent TB prior to taking medications that can reduce immunity and should be treated if found to be positive.

Nine Months Later

Tobiah had successfully completed treatment for tuberculosis disease. The local health department had done contact tracing to locate all the people he had come in close contact with before he was diagnosed, and none of them were positive for tuberculosis. On the other hand, they were able to trace the source patient who Tobiah contracted the disease from and that individual also received treatment.

What lessons have you learned, and what steps are you willing to take to improve your health?

....
....
....
....
....
....
....
....
....
....
....

....
....
....
....
....
....

SECTION 2

Other Communicable Diseases of Interest

CHAPTER 11

Ebola

Introduction: Ebola virus disease occurs in wild animals and can spread to humans and from person to person. More than half of the infected people die. The name Ebola originated from the "Ebola River," close to a village in the Democratic Republic of Congo. This village was one of the two places where Ebola first occurred in 1976. In the 2014–2016 Ebola virus disease outbreak, over 27,000 people were infected and there were over 10,000 deaths.

Types: There are five known species of Ebola virus, however the Zaire Ebola virus was responsible for the 2014–2016 outbreak.

Transmission: Humans get infected with Ebola virus when they come in contact with blood, organs, and body fluids of infected animals such as monkeys, chimpanzees, gorillas, fruit bats, forest antelope, and porcupines. Infected humans then transmit the disease to others by direct contact of their blood or body secretions with broken skin or mucus membranes of unaffected people. The people most easily infected are close contacts of those with the disease, such as household members and healthcare workers. It could take between two to twenty-one days from the time of infection to manifestation of symptoms. Once people develop symptoms, they can infect others and the virus may persist in them for up to nine months following recovery from symptoms.

Symptoms: Fever, weakness, headache, sore throat, muscle pain, vomiting, diarrhea, rash, bleeding.

Diagnosis: Laboratory testing done on the blood or oral fluid can be used to diagnose Ebola virus disease.

Treatment:
Rehydration and treatment of symptoms. Studies are still being done to find a cure for the disease, but several promising vaccines are now available for prevention.

Complications:
Damage to the kidney, damage to the liver, blood loss leading to low blood count.

Prevention:
- A vaccine was developed and used in Guinea with promising results; further research is still being done in the area of vaccine development.
- Avoid contact with animals known to spread the disease when they are ill or found dead in the wild.
- Gloves, protective clothing, goggles, and masks should be worn when taking care of infected people, and hands should be washed regularly. Laboratory testing is needed to determine when survivors become free of the virus.
- People who die from the disease should be promptly, safely, and respectfully buried.
- Close contacts of infected people should be observed for twenty-one days to ensure that they are free from the disease, thereby preventing further spread. This quarantine method helped to prevent the spread of the disease in Nigeria during the 2014–2016 outbreak in Africa.

What lessons have you learned, and what steps are you willing to take to improve your health?

CHAPTER 12

Influenza

Influenza, also known as the "flu," is a respiratory disease caused by influenza virus, mainly A and B types. It is very infectious and can be spread rapidly from person to person. Influenza occurs in seasonal epidemics (occurring in one or several regions) causing about 250,000 deaths annually. It can also occur in pandemics (occurring all over the world) such as in 1918 and in 2009. The influenza viruses have the ability to change and make themselves more infectious, hence the need for repeated annual vaccinations.

Types: Influenza A (e.g., H1N1) influenza affects both humans and animals. Influenza B affects only humans. Influenza C is a less common type.

Causes:
When an infected person coughs or sneezes, they release very tiny respiratory droplets that contain thousands of viruses that can enter the mouth or nose of people nearby. These viruses then enter into the cells of the respiratory system and cause infection. This infection leads to inflammation and destruction of cells in the respiratory system, allowing coinfections by other organisms such as bacteria. Inflammation of the respiratory system then leads to coughing and sneezing, which further spreads the disease to other healthy individuals.

Symptoms: Fever, cough, nasal discharge, headache, joint pain, muscle pain, malaise (feeling unwell), sore throat. Symptoms may last for up to two weeks before resolving.

Diagnosis:
Throat swabs and blood testing can help to detect the virus and confirm infections.

Treatment:
Supportive treatment with medications to reduce fever, adequate hydration, treatment of any superimposing bacterial infection and antivirus medications.

Complications:
Pneumonia, respiratory compromise, and death in severe cases.

Prevention:
- To avoid spreading the virus, cover your mouth and nose when coughing and sneezing.
- Practice good hand hygiene by washing hands regularly with soap and water.
- Medications are available in some countries to prevent severe disease if infection occurs.
- Vaccines are usually given seasonally and are modified to protect against possible changes in the virus, partly based on analysis of samples collected from infected people.

What lessons have you learned, and what steps are you willing to take to improve your health?

....

....

....

....

....

SECTION 3

Understanding the Connection

CHAPTER 13

Total Health

According to the World Health Organization, "Health is a state of complete physical, mental, and social well-being and not merely the absence of disease or infirmity." It is therefore possible for an individual to have no physical illness but still be unhealthy, and this understanding has contributed to the emergence of the concept of "total health."

Total health has several aspects, which are all related and have the common goal of maintaining the health and wellness of an individual. Total health includes spiritual health, physical health, emotional health, mental health, social health, and financial health.

As Christians, we are the light of the world and the salt of the earth (Matthew 5:13, 14). We should be an example to the world, displaying all-around good health. God wants us to prosper in every area of our lives, including our soul, body, and finances (3 John 1:2). The various components of total health can be grouped under: soul prosperity, physical prosperity, and financial prosperity. So where do we start? "But seek first His kingdom and His righteousness, and all these things will be given to you as well" (Matthew 6:33).

Soul Prosperity:

As believers, our manual is the Bible. It teaches us about our origin and how to live a full life. It also gives us various examples of different life choices and their results. It has been said that "experience is the best teacher," however, a wise person will also learn from the experiences of others. The foundation of our Christian life is faith. Faith is confidence in what we hope for and assurance about what we do not see (Hebrews 11:1). We are children of God through our faith in Jesus Christ (Galatians 3:26). How then do we build our faith? By hearing the Word of God (Romans 10:17). We should meditate constantly on the Bible to increase our faith and our knowledge about things of God. It is only the truth you know that can set you free (John 8:32) and this knowledge will keep you from perishing (Hosea 4:6).

People who do not take harmful substances like illicit drugs, alcohol, and cigarettes due to their religious beliefs are spared from the harmful health effects that result from these things. Membership in a church gives one a sense of community and this is a very useful support system for dealing with various situations in life.

Physical Prosperity:

To prosper physically we should eat healthy, work healthy, exercise, and interact healthily with our environment.

Eating Healthy: Food is good, but when eaten wrong it can become poison to the body.

Be intentional about your diet and plan your meals. A balanced diet is a meal that contains all the essential food nutrients in the right amounts. Poor nutrition can lead to reduced immunity, increasing an individual's chances of developing diseases. Ensure that you know the source of the food you eat. If you are dining in a restaurant, observe that it is a clean environment to reduce the chances of getting food-borne illnesses like cholera, salmonella, or hepatitis A.

Excessive food intake leads to obesity, which has become a significant problem in the world today. Obesity leads to the development of chronic diseases like diabetes and hypertension. It is also responsible for thousands of deaths. It leads to abnormal storage of fat in several organs in the body, including the liver, causing a condition called "fatty liver" that can lead to liver cancer. The basic principle of weight gain is this: the body uses up the energy it needs from the food we eat and stores the rest in the body as fat. If you are overweight, meaning that you have a BMI greater than 24.9 (BMI is calculated by dividing your weight in kilograms by the square of your height in meters kg/m^2), it is very likely that you are eating more than you need. This problem is further compounded by lack of exercise.

Dietary supplements and vitamins should be taken with caution, as when they are taken in excess, they could also cause problems. The case is also true with salt: excessive intake of salt can lead to cardiovascular diseases like hypertension and heart attack. According to WHO, salt intake can be reduced by limiting the amount of salt added in cooking to a total maximum amount "a fifth of a teaspoon" over the course of a day, reading food labels when buying processed food to check salt levels, asking for products with less salt when buying prepared food, removing salt dispensers and bottled sauces from dining tables, limiting frequent consumption of high salt products (such as salted nuts and chips), and guiding children's taste buds through a diet of mostly unprocessed foods without adding salt.

Fruits and vegetables are good but should also be eaten with moderation. There is no "one size fits all," meaning that people should eat based on their health needs. For example, someone who has high blood pressure would benefit from eating bananas, as they have potassium that help to lower the blood pressure. On the other hand someone who has uncontrolled diabetes should be careful not to eat too many bananas to avoid causing further elevation in the blood sugar level. Similarly, kiwi helps to promote good eyesight and cranberries help to prevent urinary tract infection. People with osteoporosis would benefit from eating kale, as it is a good source of calcium.

The bottom line is that to be purposeful about your health you should search out information from reliable sources about how to tailor your meals to your specific health needs.

Vaccinations: Vaccinations are beneficial to prevent various vaccine preventable diseases. Several vaccines are given from childhood into adulthood. Some vaccines that were given in childhood require booster doses in adulthood to enhance immunity to the diseases they prevent, such as diphtheria vaccine. After a vaccine is produced, vaccination surveillance is done to detect and find remedies to adverse effects that occur from the vaccines. Since the development of vaccines, they have helped to prevent millions of deaths and continue to do so.

Exercise: Exercise helps to prevent depression and several other diseases like diabetes, hypertension, heart disease, fatty liver, and obesity. It also enhances mental clarity. It is recommended that exercise should be done for at least thirty to forty minutes a day on most days or five times a week. Exercise can take several forms including walking, running, bicycling, swimming, or dancing. Any exercise is better than no exercise, so if you are unable to exercise for forty minutes, do the best you can.

Environmental Health: Ensure the cleanliness of your environment to ensure you stay healthy. Avoid overcrowding, as diseases spread very rapidly in overcrowded areas. If you live in an area where mosquitos are an issue, remove all sources of standing water from your environment as the mosquito larva thrives in stagnant water.

If you live in an area with high ozone levels, stay indoors on "ozone action days" as much as possible especially for people with respiratory diseases like asthma. Be purposeful about understanding the peculiarities of your environment and how you can live a full and healthy life in that environment.

Social Health

To be socially healthy, it is necessary to identify your support system. There is a common saying that "no man is an island" and this is true. God is the greatest support a believer has and He has graciously given us other human beings to help support us. "Two are better than one, because they have a good return for their labor: If either of them falls down, one can help the other up. But pity anyone who falls and has no one to help them up" (Ecclesiastes 4:9, 10, NIV).

Family can be a great support system. Also, friends and community members can support one another. We should regularly appreciate the people that God has placed in our lives to support us. The law of sowing and reaping works beyond crop science; it works in every area of life. If you feel like you don't have any support system, become a support person to someone and you will reap a harvest of support from other people.

Mental and Emotional Health:

"A cheerful heart is good medicine, but a crushed spirit dries up the bones" (Proverbs 17:22).

There is a form of heart disease called "Takotsubo cardiomyopathy" or "stress cardiomyopathy," that occurs due to emotional stress, and it can lead to heart failure. The Bible tells us not to be anxious. "Do not be anxious about anything, but in every situation, by prayer and petition, with thanksgiving, present your requests to God" (Philippians 4:6). God cares for us and wants us to cast all our cares on Him (1 Peter 5:7).

Life is as good as you make it. You can choose to be grateful for the things you have or to complain about the things you don't have. Money does not bring the kind of happiness that people think it does. I have met people who have several million dollars and are still unhappy. So if you were postponing your happiness until you became a millionaire, you might as well become happy now. Money does not guarantee happiness, and if not managed well, it can even create more stress and anxiety.

Nobody likes to be around complainers because they drain the energy out of their environment. If you keep complaining, one day you will look around and realize that you are all alone. God does not like people to complain. Happiness is a choice, meaning that regardless of your circumstances, you can choose to be happy. Manage time wisely. Don't waste your time or the time of others. Be purposeful about your time and remember to plan your rest.

Financial Prosperity

To prosper financially we should put God in charge over all areas of our lives including our finances. If we understand that everything we have, including our lives, comes from God we would not withhold ourselves and our resources from Him. We should pay our tithes and give our offerings to Him so that He will rebuke the devourer on our behalf (Malachi 3:8–10). We should also pay our taxes (Matthew 22:21). We should also be generous and take care of the poor and needy. If you give generously, you will also receive generously (2 Corinthians 9:6). We should show kindness to the poor, and God will repay us (Proverbs 19:17).

Don't live above your means, and as much as possible, do not live in debt. A borrower is slave to the lender (Proverbs 22:7). Having a budget helps with planning and gives you control over your money; you tell your money where to go. Seek out wise counsel from people who have genuine financial success. Learn to invest wisely. Investment is a means of making your money work for you.

Most importantly, we should focus more on storing our treasures in Heaven, as our time in eternity is far longer than our time on earth (Matthew 6:19–21).

Tying it all together

When John was a little boy, his parents were not millionaires, but they worked hard to provide for him and his siblings. John was a very happy boy and he did well in school. As he grew up he began to associate with people who were very materialistic and he stopped being grateful for the blessings in his life because he wanted to be materially wealthy. He worked very hard and paid no attention to his diet or his health. He had alienated himself from his family and surrounded himself with friends he did not trust. He was dealing with depression but assured himself that when he became a millionaire he would be happy. Within ten years, he made his first million but he was not happy at all. In fact, at this point he started taking medications for depression, diabetes, and hypertension. He had not paid much attention to his diet and had tripled his weight in ten years. He bought a very expensive sports car but was too big to fit into it so he just left it in his garage. He continued to expand his financial empire and the more he made, the sadder he got because he felt so empty. He wished he could go back to the time when he was a happy little boy. John was very down and sad despite taking maximum doses of antidepressants.

One day, he walked to the grocery store on his street and saw "Happy" Paul who had been working there for almost three years. John had seen him several times and even ignored a couple of Paul's greetings on purpose, just to annoy him. Paul never seemed bothered by anything. John was secretly jealous of Paul. Everyone seemed to like him and he was about to be married to a very happy lady—Mary. John decided to talk to Paul for the first time. He asked him if he was taking "happy" pills. This made Paul smile. Paul then went on to tell John about the love of Jesus and how it was not too late for John to accept the love of Christ. John seemed to think about it for a while, and then told Paul that he had been born into a Christian home but never had the kind of "personal relationship with Jesus" that Paul talked about. He then asked Paul what he could do. Paul told him to repent of all his bad ways and accept Jesus Christ into his heart.

Six Months Later

John had given his life to Jesus Christ and had joined the church in the community where Paul and Mary attended. He and Paul had become very close friends. They had started working out together, and Paul had encouraged John to change his diet. John had also reunited with his family. He had donated several millions of dollars to build a park in the community, where people could exercise. John had even lost most of his excess weight and had been taken off most of his medications by his doctor, as his depression, diabetes, and hypertension had all improved significantly. Best of all, John had become an evangelist, telling everyone about the love and hope that can be found in Jesus.

What lessons have you learned, and what steps are you willing to take to improve your health?

REFERENCES

1. https://www.biblegateway.com
2. www.cdc.gov
3. www.who.int
4. https://www.nhlbi.nih.gov
5. https://www.cancer.gov
6. https://www.ncbi.nlm.nih.gov

APPRECIATION

I would like to express my sincere gratitude to the Almighty God, my creator and my sustainer. I would also like to appreciate my parents, Elder Emmanuel Dyboh and Elder Abigail Dyboh, and my sisters for all their unconditional love, support, and encouragement, including their support in my years of medical school and residency.

I am grateful to my husband Emeka Ama and our children for all of their love and understanding—you guys are the best team ever!

I sincerely thank my brother, Evangelist Chidi Okeke, for encouraging me to start and finish this book. I also thank my uncle Rev, Onuka Okereke, for keeping my zeal to educate people about their health alive.

My sincere gratitude goes to Dr. Chip Carson who has been invaluable to my growth in the field of medicine and who painstakingly edited the manuscript of this book.

I thank the leaders and members of Presbyterian Church of Nigeria Okokomaiko Parish, Lagos Nigeria; the leaders and members of Grace Church, Humble, Texas; and the leaders and members of the Redeemed Christian Church of God, The King's Palace, Katy, Texas for their encouragement.

I sincerely thank everyone who has encouraged me in one way or the other. My prayer is that the seed of encouragement you have sown into my life would produce bountiful blessings for you. Amen.

ABOUT THE AUTHOR

Ifeoma Margaret Ama MD., MPH, has been practicing medicine for over a decade and currently practices in Houston Texas, where she lives with her family. She specializes in Family Medicine and Occupational Medicine. She is very passionate about educating people about their health and teaching them ways to stay healthy, which prompted her to obtain a masters degree in Public Health. In the course of her medical career, she has been the recipient of several excellence awards. Her greatest joy however, is knowing the love and mercy of God and sharing this message with people.

www.ingramcontent.com/pod-product-compliance
Lightning Source LLC
Chambersburg PA
CBHW031153250726
48655CB00002B/949